PROMISING MARIJUANA AND CBD MEDICAL TREATMENTS

Mickey Dee

Copyright © 2018 by Mickey Dee

All rights reserved. No part of this book can be reproduced without the prior permission of the author and publisher.

Disclaimer: This book is sold with the understanding that the author and publisher are not medical professionals and are not engaged in offering medical advice. The purpose of this book is to compliment and supplement other texts on the subject. You are urged to read all available information, consult your doctor and learn as much as possible before starting any treatment. Every effort has been made to make the book as accurate as possible. Use this book as a general guide and be sure to check the laws and regulations in your area. The author and publisher shall have no liability or responsibility to any person or entity with respect to any loss or damage caused or alleged to be causes, directly or indirectly by the information contained in this book. The book is not affiliated with any government.

Table of Contents

Introduction 1

What Is Medical Marijuana? 6

Everything You Need To Know About CBD Oil 13

Cannabis Cure? What You Weed To Know About CBD Oil 24

Medical Marijuana 53

CBD: Medicine From Marijuana 60

Marijuana Cancer Treatment 79

Cannabis And Cancer: How "Marijuana" Helps The Body Heal 87

Cancer: Can Cannabis Really Cure It? 99

Marijuana And Cancer 104

Medical Marijuana And Anxiety Disorders 126

One Can Conclude 138

Introduction

Cannabis, also known as marijuana among other names, is a psychoactive drug from the Cannabis plant intended for medical or recreational use. The main psychoactive part of cannabis is tetrahydrocannabinol (THC), one of 483 known compounds in the plant, including at least 65 other cannabinoids. Cannabis can be used by smoking, vaporizing, within food, or as an extract.

Cannabis is often used for its mental and physical effects, such as a "high" or stoned" feeling, a general change in perception, heightened mood, and an increase in appetite. Onset of effects is within minutes when smoked, and about 30 to 60 minutes when cooked and eaten. They last for between two and six hours. Short-term side effects may include a decrease in short-term memory, dry mouth, impaired motor skills, red eyes, and feelings of paranoia or anxiety. Long-term side effects may include addiction, decreased mental ability in those who started as teenagers, and behavioral problems in children whose mothers used cannabis during pregnancy. Studies have found a strong relation between cannabis use and the risk of psychosis, though the cause-and-effect relationship is debated.

Medical cannabis, or medical marijuana, can refer to the use of cannabis and its cannabinoids to treat disease or improve symptoms; however, there is no single agreed-upon definition. The rigorous scientific study of cannabis as a medicine has been hampered by production restrictions and other federal regulations. There is limited evidence suggesting cannabis can be used to reduce nausea and vomiting during chemotherapy, to improve appetite in people with HIV/AIDS, and to treat chronic pain and muscle spasms. Its use for other medical applications is insufficient for conclusions about safety or efficacy.

Short-term use increases the risk of both minor and major adverse effects. Common side effects include dizziness, feeling tired and vomiting. Long-term effects of cannabis are not clear. Concerns include memory and cognition problems, risk of addiction, schizophrenia in young people, and the risk of children taking it by accident.

Cannabis has psychoactive and physiological effects when consumed. The immediate desired effects from consuming cannabis include relaxation and euphoria (the "high" or "stoned" feeling), a general alteration of conscious perception, increased awareness of sensation, increased libido and distortions in the perception of time and space. At higher doses, effects can include altered body image, auditory and/or visual illusions, pseudohallucinations and ataxia from selective impairment of polysynaptic reflexes. In some cases, cannabis can lead to dissociative states such as depersonalization and derealization.

Some immediate undesired side effects include a decrease in short-term memory, dry mouth, impaired motor skills and reddening of the eyes. Aside from a subjective change in perception and mood, the most common short-term physical and neurological effects include increased heart rate, increased appetite and consumption of food, lowered blood pressure, impairment of short-term and working memory, psychomotor coordination, and concentration. Some users may experience an episode of acute psychosis, which usually abates after six hours, but in rare instances, heavy users may find the symptoms continuing for many days. A reduced quality of life is associated with heavy cannabis use, although the relationship is inconsistent and weaker than for tobacco and other substances. It is unclear, however, if the relationship is cause and effect.

What Is Medical Marijuana?

Medical marijuana is any part of the marijuana plant that you use to treat health problems. People use it to get relief from their symptoms, not to try to get high.

Most marijuana that's sold legally as medicine has the same ingredients as the kind that people use for pleasure. But some medical marijuana is specially grown to have less of the chemicals that cause feelings of euphoria.

Ingredients in Medical Marijuana

Marijuana plants have multiple chemicals, known as

cannabinoids. The two main ones are THC and CBD. THC gives some of the pleasurable effects that pot smokers are looking for, but it also has some effects that may treat medical problems.

Some research suggests that CBD may be helpful for some health issues, but it doesn't cause you to get high.

How Marijuana Works on the Brain?

People who smoke marijuana begin to feel its effects almost immediately, while those who eat it may not feel it for up to an hour.

When you smoke pot, THC goes from your lungs to the bloodstream and causes your brain cells to release the chemical dopamine, leaving you feeling high.

Experts know less about how CBD works. They think it may work sometimes with THC, and sometimes on its own, to have an effect on the brain.

Uses for Medical Marijuana

Medical marijuana may help ease pain, nausea, and loss of appetite in people who have cancer and HIV. There's not a lot of research on these areas yet, though.

Some research suggests medical marijuana may cut down seizures in people with epilepsy. Some studies show it also may ease multiple sclerosis symptoms like muscle stiffness and spasms, pain, and frequent urination.

Short-Term Side Effects

Medical marijuana can change your mood, making you feel happy, relaxed, sleepy, or anxious. It can also disrupt your short-term memory and decision-making ability. These side effects can last 1 to 3 hours.

Large doses of medical marijuana can make some people have hallucinations, delusions, and paranoia. Research suggests that smoking marijuana can make breathing problems, like bronchitis, worse.

Long-Term Side Effects

Regular smokers of medical marijuana may get respiratory problems, such as a daily cough and a higher risk of lung infections.

Studies also link routine use to mental illness, depression, anxiety, less motivation, and suicidal thoughts among young people. Marijuana use during pregnancy can raise the risk of health problems in babies. Marijuana use can result in addiction.

Drugs Made From Marijuana

The FDA has approved two drugs that include ingredients also found in marijuana. Dronabinol has synthetic THC and is used to treat nausea from chemotherapy and extreme weight loss in AIDs patients.

Nabilone is used for the same reasons, but it has a man-made chemical that's similar to THC.

Forms of Medical Marijuana

Users smoke medical marijuana in paper-rolled cigarettes or pipes. You can also brew it into a beverage, eat it in cooked foods, or take it in pill form. The effects of a marijuana pill can be strong and long-lasting. This makes it hard to predict how it will affect a person. It can also be inhaled through vaporizers. Cannabinoid receptors have also been found in skin. Some use topical marijuana for pain and inflammation. More research is needed.

Where Medical Marijuana Is Legal

California voters were the first to legalize medical marijuana, in 1996. It's now legal in almost half of U.S. states.

If you live in a state where it's legal and your doctor has OK'd it, you can buy it from an authorized seller known as a dispensary. Some people may legally grow their own medical marijuana.

Medical Marijuana for Children

Some studies suggest medical marijuana may help relieve seizures in children with hard-to-treat epilepsy.

A type of medical marijuana known as "Charlotte's Web" may help kids without getting them high, because the strain has very little THC.

Everything You Need To Know About CBD Oil

People take or apply cannabidiol to treat a variety of symptoms, but its use is controversial. There is some confusion about what it is and the effects it has on the human body.

Cannabidiol (CBD) may have some health benefits, and it may also pose risks. Products containing the compound are now legal in many American states where marijuana is not.

What is CBD oil?

CBD is one of many compounds, known as

cannabinoids, in the cannabis plant. Researchers have been looking at the potential therapeutic uses of CBD.

Oils that contain concentrations of CBD are known as CBD oils. The concentrations and the uses of these oils vary.

Is CBD marijuana?

CBD oil is a cannabinoid derived from the cannabis plant.

Until recently, the best-known compound in cannabis was delta-9 tetrahydrocannabinol (THC). This is the most active ingredient in marijuana.

Marijuana contains both THC and CBD, and these compounds have different effects.

Marijuana contains both THC and CBD, and these compounds have different effects.

THC creates a mind-altering "high" when it is broken down by heat and introduced into the body. This results from smoking marijuana or using it in cooking, for example.

Unlike THC, CBD is not psychoactive. This means that it does not change the state of mind of the person who uses it.

However, CBD does appear to produce significant changes in the body, and some research suggests that it has medical benefits.

The least processed form of the cannabis plant, known as hemp, contains most of the CBD used medicinally. Though hemp and marijuana come from the same plant, Cannabis sativa, the two are very different.

Over the years, marijuana farmers have selectively bred their plants to contain high levels of THC and other compounds that interested them, often because the compounds produced a smell or had another effect on the plant's flowers.

However, hemp farmers have rarely modified the plant. These hemp plants are used to create CBD oil.

How CBD works

All cannabinoids, including CBD, produce effects in the body by attaching to certain receptors.

The human body produces certain cannabinoids on its own. It also has two receptors for cannabinoids, called the CB1 receptors and CB2 receptors.

CB1 receptors are located throughout the body, but many are in the brain.

The CB1 receptors in the brain deal with coordination and movement, pain, emotions, and mood, thinking, appetite, and memories, among other factors. THC attaches to these receptors.

CB2 receptors are more common in the immune system. They affect inflammation and pain.

Researchers once believed that CBD attached to these CB2 receptors, but it now appears that CBD does not attach directly to either receptor. Instead, it seems to direct the body to use more of its own cannabinoids.

Benefits

Because of the way that CBD acts in the body, it has many potential benefits.

Natural pain relief and anti-inflammatory properties
People tend to use prescription or over-the-counter drugs to relieve stiffness and pain, including chronic pain.

Quitting smoking and drug withdrawals

Some promising evidence suggests that CBD use may help people to quit smoking. A pilot study published in Addictive Behaviors found that smokers who used inhalers containing CBD smoked fewer cigarettes than usual and had no further cravings for nicotine.

A similar review, published in Neurotherapeutics found that CBD may be a promising treatment for people with opioid addiction disorders.

The researchers noted that CBD reduced some symptoms associated with substance use disorders.

These included anxiety, mood-related symptoms, pain, and insomnia.

More research is necessary, but these findings suggest that CBD may help to prevent or reduce withdrawal symptoms.

Epilepsy

After researching the safety and effectiveness of CBD oil for treating epilepsy, the FDA approved the use of CBD (Epidiolex) as a therapy for two rare conditions characterized by of epileptic seizures.

In the U.S., a doctor can prescribe Epidiolex to treat:

Lennox-Gastaut syndrome (LGS), a condition that appears between the ages of 3 and 5 years and involves different kinds of seizures

Dravet syndrome (DS), a rare genetic condition that appears in the first year of life and involves frequent, fever-related seizures

The types of seizures that characterize LGS or DS are difficult to control with other types of medication.

The FDA specified that doctors could not prescribe Epidiolex for children younger than 2 years. A physician or pharmacist will determine the right dosage based on body weight.

Other neurological symptoms and disorders

Researchers are studying the effects of CBD on various neuropsychiatric disorders.

Review noted that CBD has anti-seizure properties and a low risk of side effects for people with epilepsy.

Studies suggest that CBD may also treat many complications linked to epilepsy, such as neurodegeneration, neuronal injury, and psychiatric diseases.

Another study, published in Current Pharmaceutical Design, found that CBD may produce effects similar to those of certain antipsychotic drugs, and that the compound may provide a safe and effective treatment for people with schizophrenia.

Fighting cancer

Some researchers have found that CBD may prove to combat cancer.

Authors of a review published in the British Journal of Clinical Pharmacology found evidence that CBD significantly helped to prevent the spread of cancer.

In addition, the researchers noted that the compound tends to suppress the growth of cancer cells and promote their destruction.

The authors pointed out that CBD has low levels of toxicity and called for further research into its potential as an accompaniment to standard cancer treatments.

Anxiety disorders

Doctors often advise people with chronic anxiety to avoid cannabis, as THC can trigger or amplify feelings of anxiousness and paranoia.

However, authors of a review from Neurotherapeutics found that CBD may help to reduce anxiety in people with certain related disorders.

According to the review, CBD may reduce anxiety-related behaviors in people with conditions such as:

- post-traumatic stress disorder

- general anxiety disorder

- panic disorder

- social anxiety disorder

- obsessive-compulsive disorder

The authors noted that current treatments for these disorders can lead to additional symptoms and side effects, which can cause some people to stop taking them.

Cannabis Cure? What You Weed To Know About CBD Oil

At Eats of Eden health food store in Limerick, staff were keeping a close eye on the global cannabis trend. They could see that cannabidiol was making huge waves in the US and Canada. It was seen as a legal alternative to marijuana and there were claims it was beneficial for a plethora of health problems — from epilepsy to pain, anxiety to sleep difficulties.

We knew it would ripple over to Ireland, that it would take off here," says Eats of Eden proprietor Cillín Cleere, a nutritional therapist with a degree in biochemistry and one of the first to stock it in Ireland.

Cannabidiol (CBD) is one of the major cannabinoids in the cannabis plant — out of a total of more than 110 in the plant. It's also found in hemp. CBD is not psychoactive in the same way THC is, so it won't make you high. Its pharmacology is different to THC, the principal euphoria-inducing psychoactive agent in cannabis.

Charlotte's Web is one of the most high-profile CBD oils. A high-CBD, low-THC cannabis extract, it has been on the market the longest.

Cleere isn't sure if his was the first health food store in Ireland to stock CBD oil but he says Eats of Eden "definitely got behind it in a big way". For nearly two years now, it's been selling Swiss, Northern Irish, and Irish-made CBD oil products, with prices ranging from €18 to €73, depending on strength/volume of the individual product.

Feedback has been "incredible", he says, adding that in the store, CBD oil "probably would be the top seller at the moment".

Those who buy it span a broad demographic – "including parents who give it to their kids, busy professionals on the go, weekend warriors and athletes, and a good few pet owners. People generally come in looking for advice on immune and joint support or help with a hectic, busy lifestyle which can leave their nerves a bit frazzled."

Cleere says repeat business is pretty good.

In Ireland, CBD is not illegal under the Misuse of Drugs Act. But neither is it a recognised, legal medicine approved by the Health Products Regulatory Authority.

In Ireland, we can buy CBD so long as it contains less than 0.2% THC. People can buy it online, in health food stores, and in some pharmacies. They can use it legally.

So why would you buy it? Finn points to a top three of disorders where the greatest weight of evidence for CBD benefit currently exists. "Inflammatory pain is one of the key disorders that CBD has been proposed for — such as low back pain and arthritic pain. Another key disorder where there is some published evidence for efficacy is childhood epilepsy. And there's some limited evidence that CBD could be useful for psychiatric disorders including anxiety disorders.

New England Journal of Medicine carried news of a trial of CBD for drug-resistant seizures in Dravet syndrome — complex childhood epilepsy. It found CBD resulted in a greater reduction in convulsive-seizure frequency than placebo. And a review published in the journal Neurotherapeutics found evidence from human studies "strongly supports the potential for CBD as a treatment for anxiety disorders". This review emphasised the "potential value and need for further study" of CBD in treatment of anxiety.

It has also been used in certain forms of arthritis, Parkinson's disease, and migraine. But I'd like to see patients taking it under the care of a consultant with a special interest."

Cleere says the huge scientific interest in cannabis was sparked by the discovery of the endocannabinoid system (ECS), a complex, fat-based network of chemical messengers and receptors that help fine-tune our biochemistry, keeping us healthy and strong.

All animals have an ECS — ours helps regulate appetite, pain and stress levels. It balances mood and memory and keeps our immune system in tip-top shape. We now know a diet lacking in vitamins, minerals, and omegas, along with eating processed foods, prolonged stress and exposure to harmful chemicals all contribute towards weakened ECS. When this happens, illness occurs, a phenomenon referred to as endocannabinoid deficiency syndrome," explains Cleere.

Many plants make molecules identical to our own ECS messengers that can directly nourish a weakened ECS system. "The cannabis family has the highest concentration of these nourishing molecules known as cannabinoids, which include THC and CBD. Other food sources include Echinacea, black pepper, and dark chocolate. Small amounts of cannabinoid-rich foods and oils contribute towards healthy ECS.

cannabis plant is complex. Alongside its 110-plus cannabinoids, it also has 700 other molecules. "Oils prepared from the plant will usually contain other molecules and components [besides cannabidiol] and it's currently uncertain to what extent these other molecules contribute to the pharmacological effect of the oil."

Some CBD oils will contain significant amounts of cannabidiol, but adds there's huge variability among the different oils and some of the preparations may have too much or too little cannabidiol. "The oils can vary from batch to batch, from seller to seller. What you buy in a pharmacy in Cork could be very different to what you might buy in a health food store in Galway."

Consumers are recommends to try and understand the contents, purity, and quality of what they're taking. "Very few of the oils that you can buy on the market have been tested rigorously in clinical trials.

If you buy it from reputable health food stores, it should have undergone the necessary quality assurance tests to ensure it complies with required minimal THC levels.

CBD definitely has health benefits but it's not a panacea. It won't help with everything. A lot of misleading claims have been made about it.

He sees a good benefit in its anti-inflammatory effect and in the fact there are no reports of it harming health. In this way, it's perhaps superior to ibuprofen, which can cause digestive problems. "If it presents an alternative to non-steroidal anti- inflammatory drugs, it's worth investigating."

However, he cautions that the amounts of cannabidiol people buy in CBD oils tend to be low. "How much is a pharmacological effect and how much placebo is up for debate.

CBD appears to be generally well-tolerated, some people have reported side-effects that include gastrointestinal symptoms like diarrhoea, vomiting, and nausea. Other side-effects can include dizziness, fatigue, and sedation. CBD can affect how other drugs are metabolised in the body, so it's important to liaise with your doctor if taking prescribed medicine.

What is CBD? The 'miracle' cannabis compound that doesn't get you high

The cannabis-derived chemical is non-psychoactive, and – while federally illegal – has been hailed as a cure for disease.

In early May, a federal court declined to protect cannabidiol (CBD), a chemical produced by the cannabis plant, from federal law enforcement, despite widespread belief in its medical value.

The ruling was contrary to existing evidence, which suggests the chemical is safe and could have multiple important uses as medicine. Many cannabis advocates consider it a miracle medicine, capable of relieving conditions as disparate as depression, arthritis and diabetes.

The perception of its widespread medical benefits have made the chemical a rallying cry for legalization advocates.

The first thing to know about CBD is that it is not psychoactive; it doesn't get people high. The primary psychoactive ingredient in marijuana is tetrahydrocannabinol (THC). But THC is only one of the scores of chemicals – known as cannabinoids – produced by the cannabis plant.

So far, CBD is the most promising compound from both a marketing and a medical perspective. Many users believe it helps them relax, despite it not being psychoactive, and some believe regular doses help stave off Alzheimer's and heart disease.

Expots: medical marijuana draws parents to US for their children's treatments.

While studies have shown CBD to have anti-inflammatory, anti-pain and anti-psychotic properties, it has seen only minimal testing in human clinical trials, where scientists determine what a drug does, how much patients should take, its side effects and so on.

Despite the government ruling, CBD is widely available over the counter in dispensaries in states where marijuana is legal.

CBD first came to public attention in a 2013 CNN documentary called Weed. The piece, reported by Dr

Sanjay Gupta, featured a little girl in Colorado named Charlotte, who had a rare life-threatening form of epilepsy called Dravet syndrome.

At age five, Charlotte suffered 300 grand mal seizures a week, and was constantly on the brink of a medical emergency. Through online research, Charlotte's desperate parents heard of treating Dravet with CBD. It was controversial to pursue medical marijuana for such a young patient, but when they gave Charlotte oil extracted from high-CBD cannabis, her seizures stopped almost completely. In honor of her progress, high-CBD cannabis is sometimes known as Charlotte's Web.

CBD has been sought for its healing properties.

Facebook Twitter Pinterest CBD has been sought for its healing properties.

Illustration: George Wylesol

After Charlotte's story got out, hundreds of families relocated to Colorado where they could procure CBD for their children, though not all experienced such life- changing results. Instead of moving, other families obtained CBD oil through the illegal distribution networks.

In late June, the US Food and Drug Administration could approve the Epidiolex, a pharmaceuticalized form of CBD for several severe pediatric seizure disorders. According to data recently published in the New England Journal of Medicine, the drug can reduce seizures by more than 40%. If Epidiolex wins approval it would be the first time the agency approves a drug derived from the marijuana plant. (The FDA has approved synthetic THC to treat chemotherapy-related nausea.)

Epidiolex was developed by the London-based GW Pharmaceuticals, which grows cannabis on tightly controlled farms in the UK. It embarked on the Epidiolex project in 2013, as anecdotes of CBD's value as an epilepsy drug began emerging from the US.

While parents treating their children with CBD had to proceed based on trial and error, like a folk medicine, they also had to wonder whether dispensary purchased CBD was professionally manufactured and contained what the package said it did. GW brought a scientific understanding and pharmaceutical grade manufacturing to this promising compound.

Fortunately, like THC, CBD appears to be well tolerated; as far as we can tell, there are no recorded incidents of fatal CBD overdoses.

Since Weed first aired, GW's stock has climbed 1,500%.

Should I grow my own weed at home? Here's what you need to know GW's first drug Sativex, which contains both CBD and THC, is available as a treatment for MS-related spasticity in Canada, Australia, and much of Europe and Latin America.

The company is also studying cannabinoid-based drugs as a treatment for autism spectrum disorders, an aggressive brain tumor called glioblastoma, and schizophrenia.

Other industries, not subject to the strict regulations governing pharmaceuticals are eager to develop their own CBD products, everything from joints and vape pens to skin creams and edibles which may or may not have valid medical use.

In Los Angeles, it's among the latest wellness fads. It can be found in cocktails, and an upscale juice shop will even add a few drops of CBD infused olive oil to a beverage for $3.50.

5 Most Dangerous Diseases in the World Treated By Cannabis Oil

The true extent of CBD's healing abilities might shock you...

With medical technology further advancing with each new day that passes, there certainly seems to be plenty of hope when it comes to treating diseases, particularly rare or dangerous ones, which were earlier thought to be unstoppable. Numerous new therapies, treatment plans and medications exist to help slow down the effects of some debilitating medical conditions, but still no medically approved cure has been discovered. What the medical world might not want you to know, is that cannabis oil, sometimes labeled as CBD or cannabidiol oil, has shown great promise as a way to not only slow down some of the world's most dangerous medical conditions, but it also may act as a possible cure for them as well.

Of course, widespread publication of this information to the general public would not only bankrupt big pharma, chances are it would put certain medical practitioners out of business too. Nevertheless, it is vital to stay informed, especially in this day and age where the truth is so easily accessible and in reach through the internet, as long as you are willing to keep questioning what is presented in society and through the media.

What Is Cannabis Oil, aka CBD Oil?:

Cannabis oil, typically referred to by the name CBD

oil or cannabidiol oil, is an extracted compound from the cannabis plant, with origins from both the female marijuana crop and industrial hemp. Cannabidiol is one of around 100 different cannabinoids present in the marijuana crop. It binds to the CB1 and CB2 receptors throughout the body's already present endocannabinoid system (ECS) and assists with the regular functions of this internal operation.

The body naturally produces its own cannabinoids throughout the ECS, which are referred to as endocannabinoids. Meanwhile, cannabinoids from outside sources are called phytocannabinoids. The ECS is responsible for regulating homeostasis throughout a multitude of important activities, including sleep, mood, hormones, appetite, pain sensitivity, reproductivity, fertility and more. CBD is a unique compound because it acts multi-dimensionally.

Whether the body is experiencing a surplus or a shortage of endocannabinoids throughout the ECS, cannabidiol is able to once again bring balance to the target area and restore equilibrium. For this reason, cannabidiol is truly capable of tuning in to what the body needs, listening to its requests and fulfilling its purpose where it can help, showing that in many ways this cannabinoid holds an intelligence of its own.

1. CBD helps Treat Epilepsy/Seizures:

One aspect in particular that has driven CBD oil into becoming a household term amongst cannabis consumers, is because of the profound stories reported about individuals with incurable epilepsy and seizures who saw a significant decrease in the quantity of their episodes after using the all-natural healing compound. Countless studies do exist which express cannabidiol's effectiveness, which presents a sizeable chunk of evidence that this could be the answer that those with epilepsy have been seeking.

A study published in the Journal of Pharmacological and Experimental Therapeutics, for example, displayed very promising results. During this experiment in vitro electrophysiology and an in vivo animal seizure model were both utilized to test CBD's effectiveness, and to examine whether or not it could be used as a possible anticonvulsant and antiseizure solution. The results were quite clear, with the researchers making a statement that "…these findings suggest that CBD acts, potentially in a CB(1) receptor-independent manner, to inhibit epileptiform activity in vitro and seizure severity in vivo.

Another examination, published in the Journal of Clinical Pharmacology, describes numerous comparisons of the anticonvulsant properties of cannabidiol (CBD). Although the journal goes deep into complex analysis, the ultimate released conclusion states that "…the anticonvulsant nature of cannabidiol suggests it has a therapeutic potential in at least three of the four major types of epilepsy: grand mal, cortical focal, and complex partial seizures".

There are plenty of other studies that could be referenced, but the main point to understand is that significant evidence does exist with relation to cannabidiol (CBD) and its antiepileptic, antiseizure, and anticonvulsant properties.

2. Cancer: CBD for Pain Relief

Cancer is debilitating, affecting more than 15 million individuals in the United States alone, and these are only the cases that have been diagnosed. Although many conventional medical treatments exist to diminish cancer or remove the infected cells from the body (which allows diagnosed individuals the chance for full recovery and rehabilitation), there has never been an actual cure for cancer. However, CBD oil could be a promising option. As with epilepsy and seizures, just as many (if not more) conclusive studies exist that show just how well cannabidiol has been in terms of diminishing the profligacy of cancer cells.

An article posted in the British Journal of Clinical Pharmacology not only expressed that cannabinoids had anti-tumor properties, but went as far as to claim that CBD analogues are important and worth exploring for how they can be utilized as an alternative to therapeutic agents.

Molecular Cancer Therapeutics also released a thorough account of cannabidiol's effectiveness at managing breast cancer cells, and the findings explained that CBD is capable of demolishing malignant tumors through a process involving the switching off of a specific expression of the ID-1 gene, which is a protein that is closely tied with cancer growth.

Cannabidiol is not only a noninvasive compound, it also is connected with relatively few side effects, which is why its widespread utilization for cancer treatment could be a huge development. Further research is in process which only adds to the accumulating collection of scientific evidence for CBD's link to preventing cancer cell growth.

3. HIV/AIDS:

Many new test medications have entered the market as not only a way to manage the symptoms of HIV/AIDS, but also to suppress and potentially prevent the contraction of this disease altogether.

When it first appeared in the United States in the 1980's, HIV/AIDS was a real epidemic; people were dying, and the world thought for sure there'd never be a way to stop this rampant disease from spreading.

As time went on, though, new discoveries were made and now, even though many people have been diagnosed with HIV/AIDS, this blood-borne disease is relatively manageable and preventable as long as the proper precautions are taken. Cannabis oil has also shown some promise as a means to decline the symptoms and challenges tied with HIV/AIDS.

One study in particular, released in the scientific journal "Genes & Cancer," links cannabidiol to inhibition of the growth of kaposi sarcoma neoplasms, which is prevalent amongst AIDS patients and those who have been diagnosed with HIV. The findings state, "…this suggests a potential mechanism by which CBD exerts its effects on

KSHV-infected endothelium, and supports the further examination of CBD as a novel targeted agent for the treatment of Kaposi sarcoma, Genes & Cancer.

HIV/AIDS is without a doubt one of the most dangerous diseases on this list, and the studies that have been published on CBD as a potential remedy for the condition have been positive overall. However, there simply needs to be (much) more of them – including clinical trials – in order to properly backup any claims that cannabis oil can act as a cure.

4. Amyotrophic Lateral Sclerosis (ALS):

With the massive internet craze a couple years back about the "Ice Bucket Challenge", amyotrophic lateral sclerosis or ALS gained widespread and much needed attention – setting off a wave of donations and funding for further medical research to be conducted pertaining to this condition. In addition to the conventional medical advancements being made, cannabidiol (CBD) also shows some promising results as a possible solution for slowing down the effects of ALS.

American Journal of Hospice and Palliative Care posted their research findings pertaining to the various aspects in which cannabidiol is known to have a positive affect, and how these abnormal physiological processes all tie together in the debilitating case of ALS. The study urges further clinical trials and research to be conducted, and the scientists claimed that, "…based on the currently available scientific data, it is reasonable to think that cannabis might significantly slow the progression of ALS, potentially extending life expectancy and substantially reducing the overall burden of the disease".

Considering that research has only recently blossomed pertaining to ALS, and how it affects those who are diagnosed with it, it does not come as a surprise that there is little evidence to support claims that CBD is effective at managing ALS symptoms. However, the world is urged to support further clinical trials of this possibility, because many connections seem to show promise – especially in the eyes of some top- notch scientists who can see the potential of cannabidiol for this application.

5. Multiple Sclerosis (MS): Relieving the Pain

Multiple Sclerosis, more commonly known by its shortened acronym MS, is an unpredictable disease that predominantly affects the central nervous system and its functions. It is estimated that around 400,000 individuals in the United States have been diagnosed with MS, and in many ways very little is understood about this debilitating medical condition.

One medicine in particular, known as Sativex, shows quite a lot of promise not only for managing symptoms of MS, but also for managing numerous other medical conditions as well. Sativex is the first cannabis-based medication to reach the stage of conventional clinical development, which is a massive accomplishment in the overall fight to normalize marijuana for medical purposes.

A study published in the Expert Opinion on Pharmacotherapy reviews the effectiveness of Sativex for symptoms of MS, and claims that "Sativex has been approved for use in neuropathic pain due to multiple sclerosis in Canada. If ongoing studies replicate the results already observed, further approvals for the treatment of spasticity in Multiple Sclerosis and for neuropathic pain are likely".

Sativex seems to be the most researched possibility for a reliable Multiple Sclerosis treatment, but it seems that numerous cannabinoids – including cannabidiol – seem to be effective at managing some of these debilitating symptoms. It will be interesting to see how clinical research develops over the next decade, and it is incredible that Sativex is already available for patient use in many parts of the country.

Medical Marijuana

There are few subjects that can stir up stronger emotions among doctors, scientists, researchers, policy makers, and the public than medical marijuana. Is it safe? Should it be legal? Decriminalized? Has its effectiveness been proven? What conditions is it useful for? Is it addictive? How do we keep it out of the hands of teenagers? Is it really the "wonder drug" that people claim it is? Is medical marijuana just a ploy to legalize marijuana in general?

These are just a few of the excellent questions around this subject, questions that I am going to studiously avoid so we can focus on two specific areas: why do patients find it useful, and how can they discuss it with their doctor?

Marijuana is currently legal, on the state level, in 29 states, and in Washington, DC. It is still illegal from the federal government's perspective. The Obama administration did not make prosecuting medical marijuana even a minor priority.

President Donald Trump promised not to interfere with people who use medical marijuana, though his administration is currently threatening to reverse this policy. About 85% of Americans support legalizing medical marijuana, and it is estimated that at least several million Americans currently use it.

Marijuana without the high

Least controversial is the extract from the hemp plant known as CBD (which stands for cannabidiol) because this component of marijuana has little, if any, intoxicating properties. Marijuana itself has more than 100 active components. THC (which stands for tetrahydrocannabinol) is the chemical that causes the "high" that goes along with marijuana consumption. CBD-dominant strains have little or no THC, so patients report very little if any alteration in consciousness.

Patients do, however, report many benefits of CBD, from relieving insomnia, anxiety, spasticity, and pain to treating potentially life-threatening conditions such as epilepsy. One particular form of childhood epilepsy called Dravet syndrome is almost impossible to control, but responds dramatically to a CBD-dominant strain of marijuana called Charlotte's Web. The videos of this are dramatic.

Uses of medical marijuana

The most common use for medical marijuana in the United States is for pain control. While marijuana isn't strong enough for severe pain (for example, post-surgical pain or a broken bone), it is quite effective for the chronic pain that plagues millions of Americans, especially as they age. Part of its allure is that it is clearly safer than opiates (it is impossible to overdose on and far less addictive) and it can take the place of NSAIDs such as Advil or Aleve, if people can't take them due to problems with their kidneys or ulcers or GERD.

In particular, marijuana appears to ease the pain of multiple sclerosis, and nerve pain in general. This is an area where few other options exist, and those that do, such as Neurontin, Lyrica, or opiates are highly sedating. Patients claim that marijuana allows them to resume their previous activities without feeling completely out of it and disengaged.

Along these lines, marijuana is said to be a fantastic muscle relaxant, and people swear by its ability to lessen tremors in Parkinson's disease. I have also heard of its use quite successfully for fibromyalgia, endometriosis, interstitial cystitis, and most other conditions where the final common pathway is chronic pain.

Marijuana is also used to manage nausea and weight loss, and can be used to treat glaucoma. A highly promising area of research is its use for PTSD in veterans who are returning from combat zones. Many veterans and their therapists report drastic improvement and clamor for more studies, and for a loosening of governmental restrictions on its study. Medical marijuana is also reported to help patients suffering from pain and wasting syndrome associated with HIV, as well as irritable bowel syndrome and Crohn's disease.

This is not intended to be an inclusive list, but rather to give a brief survey of the types of conditions for which medical marijuana can provide relief. As with all remedies, claims of effectiveness should be critically evaluated and treated with caution.

Talking with your doctor

Many patients find themselves in the situation of wanting to learn more about medical marijuana, but feel embarrassed to bring this up with their doctor. This is in part because the medical community has been, as a whole, overly dismissive of this issue. Doctors are now playing catch-up, and trying to keep ahead of their patients' knowledge on this issue. Other patients are already using medical marijuana, but don't know how to tell their doctors about this for fear of being chided or criticized.

The best advice for patients is to be entirely open and honest with your physicians and to have high expectations of them. Tell them that you consider this to be part of your care and that you expect them to be educated about it, and to be able to at least point you in the direction of the information you need.

Advice for doctors is that whether you are pro, neutral, or against medical marijuana, patients are embracing it, and although we don't have rigorous studies and "gold standard" proof of the benefits and risks of medical marijuana, we need to learn about it, be open-minded, and above all, be non-judgmental. Otherwise, our patients will seek out other, less reliable sources of information; they will continue to use it, they just won't tell us, and there will be that much less trust and strength in our doctor-patient relationship.

CBD: Medicine From Marijuana

The U.S. Food & Drug Administration approved Epidiolex, a new drug for treating rare seizure disorders. FDA approves many new drugs each year, but Epidiolex made headlines for two reasons: The strawberry-flavored syrup is designed to be palatable to young children, and its active pharmaceutical ingredient—cannabidiol—comes from marijuana.

Medicine from marijuana

Entrepreneurs get in on the ground floor with CBD from hemp Epidiolex isn't the first cannabinoid to be approved as a drug. Marinol (dronabinol), which is simply synthetic tetrahydrocannabinol (THC), has been used to boost the appetites of people undergoing chemotherapy since 1985. But Epidiolex is the first FDA-approved drug whose active ingredient, cannabidiol, is extracted from marijuana plants.

Cannabidiol, or CBD, has sprouted weedlike into a cultural phenomenon that's overgrown its roots in medical marijuana. Dietary supplements containing varying amounts of CBD have been touted as remedies for insomnia, anxiety, and pain. Makers of beauty products have cottoned on to the CBD craze too, spiking mascara, lip balm, and eye cream with the cannabinoid. CBD-infused water and sodas promise relaxation along with refreshment.

Unlike THC, the compound in marijuana that gets people high, CBD isn't psychoactive. What CBD actually does—and how it does it—is somewhat debatable. But scientists say there is hope to be sifted from all the hype. Dozens of clinical trials are taking place to determine if CBD is an effective treatment for an array of disorders while scientists try to figure out precisely how the compound works. Now that CBD has received FDA's blessing as a legitimate drug, the work, researchers say, is just beginning.

The therapeutic potential of cannabidiol, one of the major phytochemicals found in marijuana, was largely ignored by doctors and scientists for decades. But in recent years, its ability to treat rare seizure disorders has come to light, leading to the first FDA approval for a drug that contains cannabidiol. As scientists try to understand the mechanism of the compound and explore its possible health benefits, some worry that hype is threatening to outpace hope. Read on to learn more about this cultural phenomenon.?

Cannabidiol, or CBD, has sprouted weedlike into a cultural phenomenon that's overgrown its roots in medical marijuana. Dietary supplements containing varying amounts of CBD have been touted as remedies for insomnia, anxiety, and pain. Makers of beauty products have cottoned on to the CBD craze too, spiking mascara, lip balm, and eye cream with the cannabinoid. CBD-infused water and sodas promise relaxation along with refreshment.

Unlike THC, the compound in marijuana that gets people high, CBD isn't psychoactive. What CBD actually does—and how it does it—is somewhat debatable. But scientists say there is hope to be sifted from all the hype. Dozens of clinical trials are taking place to determine if CBD is an effective treatment for an array of disorders while scientists try to figure out precisely how the compound works. Now that

CBD has received FDA's blessing as a legitimate drug, the work, researchers say, is just beginning.

CBD'S THERAPEUTIC BEGINNINGS

Raphael Mechoulam, an organic chemist at the Hebrew University of Jerusalem, was among the first to explore the therapeutic potential of CBD. After determining the complete structure of the compound in 1963—several decades after it had first been isolated and studied by legendary organic chemists Roger Adams and Alexander R. Todd—Mechoulam's interest was piqued by anecdotal reports of cannabis as a seizure remedy in historic literature. He points to a 15th-century treatise on hashish that relates the tale of a poet who gave the substance to the son, who had epilepsy, of an important official in Baghdad. The son's seizures disappeared, but he had to take hashish for the rest of his life, according to the story.

Although anecdotal, and possibly fabricated, this story got Mechoulam thinking about CBD as a treatment for epilepsy. He set up a collaboration with a group in Brazil and started studying CBD in animal models of epilepsy with good results. Buoyed by their success, the researchers decided to conduct a small human trial.

Mechoulam isolated half a kilogram of CBD from hashish and sent it to São Paulo, Brazil, where it was used in a small study to test its effects in epilepsy. In the trial, which included 15 people with epilepsy taking antiseizure medication, eight people were given 200 to 300 mg of CBD daily for four and a half months in addition to the antiseizure medication, while seven people received a placebo. Four people in the CBD group experienced virtually no seizures during the trial, three others reported a partial improvement in their condition, and one person saw no change. The placebo group also experienced no change.

While the medical establishment failed to notice Mechoulam's study, decades later word of the results reached parents of children with two rare forms of epilepsy—Dravet syndrome and Lennox-Gastaut syndrome, which are characterized by frequent seizures that usually aren't controlled with medication. As medical marijuana became legal in a few U.S. states, these parents, and others affected by severe forms of epilepsy, sought out dispensaries that sold cannabis that was high in CBD and low in THC to treat their children's worsening seizures.

Sam Vogelstein didn't have Dravet syndrome or Lennox-Gastaut syndrome, but he was diagnosed with a hard-to-treat variant of epilepsy when he was four years old. By the time he was 11, in 2012, his parents had tried nearly two dozen medications to decrease the number of his seizures—five-to-20-second events where he'd partially lose consciousness, his eyes glazing over and his jaw slackening—which could happen as many as 100 times each day.

Sam's parents, Fred Vogelstein and Evelyn Nussenbaum, had also read the literature and anecdotal reports of CBD being used to treat seizures. They tried a tincture made from purportedly high-CBD marijuana supplied by a dispensary in California, where they live. But the supply's CBD content wasn't reliable, so sometimes it eased Sam's seizures and sometimes it didn't.

That inconsistent dosage—not to mention the challenge of obtaining the product in states with differing attitudes toward products made from marijuana—set families affected by rare forms of epilepsy on a trek to legitimize the drug. Vogelstein and Nussenbaum led the way after noticing a parenthetical note in the materials and methods section of a 2010 paper in Seizure that used CBD in an animal model of epilepsy. The researchers mentioned that GW Pharmaceuticals had provided CBD for the study. The British pharmaceutical company was already marketing Sativex, a combination of equal parts CBD and THC that's used to treat spasticity and other symptoms of multiple sclerosis. Although Sativex isn't approved in the U.S., it was approved in the U.K. in 2010, with many other countries following suit.

Epilepsy wasn't GW Pharmaceuticals' focus in 2012, Nussenbaum said in April when she spoke to the FDA panel reviewing the company's New Drug Application for a cannabidiol product. "But they had greenhouses, plant stock, labs, and they were extracting cannabidiol and other cannabis compounds regularly and systematically." Nussenbaum told the panel that she never aspired to treat Sam with cannabis.

The results were enough to garner FDA's green light, offering for the first time a treatment for Dravet syndrome. But Nicole Villas, a former chemist who has a son with the disorder and serves on the Dravet Syndrome Foundation's board of directors, notes that Epidiolex isn't a cure. Some patients, such as her son, don't respond to CBD. And others experience side effects, such as sleepiness, reduced appetite, diarrhea, and elevated liver enzymes, which can be a sign of liver damage.

But the fact that there is now a drug available for these children to try, Villas says, is a huge step forward. "To have something that's well manufactured, that's regulated, that can be given in highly consistent doses, and has an indication for Dravet syndrome is a wonderful thing.

THE SCIENCE OF CBD'S SUCCESS

CBD doesn't work in every person with a seizure disorder, and there's little definitive information about its mechanism of action. Scientists are now trying to unravel how it works to determine why some people benefit and others don't and also to figure out if it might alleviate other disorders. "The literature on potential molecular targets of CBD is very large and quite conflicted.

The scientific literature implicates at least 65 distinct molecular targets for CBD. Whalley says 50 of those targets can be ruled out when considering the concentrations of CBD required to engage them. For example, in one study in cells, CBD was administered at a concentration that's 500 times as great as what's possible to physically dose a patient with. Surprisingly, scientists have also determined that CBD doesn't bind to the active sites of the cannabinoid receptors CB1 and CB2, which is where one would expect cannabinoids to be most active.

ADVERTISEMENT

When it comes to CBD's anticonvulsant activity, "there isn't any existing data to say that a particular molecular target is implicated in CBD's effects of human epilepsies." But animal studies have given scientists a few ideas of how the compound might be working.

One plausible target is G protein-coupled receptor 55 (GPR55), which is expressed in the brain and peripheral organs. In the brain, it regulates synaptic transmission—the process that sends signaling molecules from one neuron to another. Connections between these brain cells are stronger when GPR55 is activated.

Seizures arise when neurons become overactive at transmitting signals, firing more frequently than they should. "CBD will actually block the GPR55 receptor," Whalley explains, and in doing so reduce how often the neuron fires. In a rodent model of epilepsy, animals engineered without GPR55 don't respond to CBD, whereas those with the receptor do.

Whalley also thinks that CBD might be desensitizing transient receptor potential vanilloid type 1 (TRPV1) to dampen seizures. "If you activate a TRPV1 receptor, an ion channel opens, and in the case of a brain cell, more calcium will flow into the brain cell.

That is actually counterproductive if you've got a seizure because it will make the cell more excitable." CBD seems to activate TRPV1, but it then quickly desensitizes the ion channel, effectively blocking the transport of calcium into the cell. Studies show that CBD doesn't work well in epileptic animals engineered not to express TRPV1.

Finally, CBD is also known to engage a channel that transports adenosine—an anticonvulsant compound that the body makes. It's highly plausible CBD inhibits seizures via adenosine, but more experiments are needed to prove the relationship.

These molecular targets aren't specific for a particular seizure type or syndrome. So, CBD could be used for other types of seizure disorders, including intractable epilepsy, but that the clinical work still needs to be done.

"The only really compelling clinical evidence to date is essentially the three clinical trials where we've reported results for seizure.

PROMISING PROSPECTS

Because CBD appears to be able to engage so many targets, researchers have been exploring its use for a number of diseases. Its interaction with voltage-dependent anion channel 1 hints that it might be useful for treating movement disorders, such as Parkinson's disease. And its ability to interact with serotonin receptors makes scientists think it could be useful for treating depression, anxiety, and psychosis in bipolar disorder and schizophrenia. At low concentrations, CBD can bind to an allosteric site on the endocannabinoid receptor CB1 and prevent that receptor from effectively binding to THC at its active site—a mechanism that could be used to treat disorders, such as obesity, where there's excessive activation of CB1 by cannabinoids made by our bodies.

But just because CBD interacts with those receptors doesn't mean it elicits an effect. "What's really needed is clinical data in patients. We need to see what's genuine hope and what's hype. It is much more expensive and difficult and time consuming to do human studies, but at the end of the day, that's what is needed.

Roger McIntyre, a University of Toronto psychiatrist and pharmacologist, agrees. "Broadly, the scientific basis for cannabidiol is very strong. Where things start getting a little thin is when it comes to rigorous, large, randomized, controlled trials, which are the gold standard in medicine." There are currently more than 40 active clinical trials of CBD for use as a treatment for a wide range of disorders, including cocaine dependence, Parkinson's disease, and bipolar depression.

McIntyre is particularly interested in using CBD to treat mental illness, for which existing medications often don't help. "There's not just an unmet need. There's an urgent, pressing, unmet need for something very different" from the medications currently available to treat mental illness.

And yet, when McIntyre is asked if he'd recommend using CBD to treat mental illness, his answer is a resounding no. Before he changes his answer, he wants to see more clinical data. "What's there for CBD looks very promising. At the same time, there have been many occasions in the past where what we thought was promising in theory didn't quite pan out."

CBD has a lot of potential in many different areas, but one has to be clear about what the expectation is, a pharmacologist who studies cannabinoids at Dalhousie University and executive director of the

International Cannabinoid Research Society. "The hype around it is probably pushing it to a position where we may have expectations that go beyond the evidence that we have."

Gathering that evidence, particularly in the U.S., has been a daunting enterprise. As a compound that's derived from marijuana, CBD is listed as a Schedule substance. Historically, that has limited the number of researchers that have access to it.

You need a separate license for each marijuana-based compound you study. For example, his lab had permission to study THC, but when they became interested in studying CBD, they had to apply for a separate license. A year passed before the Drug Enforcement Administration gave Roth the official nod. With obstacles like that, "you have to be pretty motivated."

Now that FDA has approved Epidiolex, DEA's scheduling of CBD will have to change. This is good news.

MARIJUANA CANCER TREATMENT

Marijuana (also known as pot, weed, Mary Jane, hash, etc.) comes from the leaves and buds of the cannabis plant. The plant's medicinal practices go back centuries, but today the plant remains controversial in the United States. The U.S. Drug Enforcement Administration has labeled marijuana a Schedule drug, which means it's illegal under federal law. But the use of medical marijuana is legal in many states. Currently, 28 states and the District of Columbia allow medical marijuana but the qualifying conditions can vary.

Marijuana

Marijuana has active ingredients called cannabinoids that can help regulate a number of biological functions in many organisms. Delta-9-tetrahydrocannabinol (THC) is a cannabinoid that produces a "high" feeling that many users attribute to marijuana, but it can also be beneficial for many side effects of cancer and its treatments. Cannabidiol (CBD) is another cannabinoid that has many potential applications in cancer and other serious medical conditions.

Cancer and Marijuana

A number of studies involving individuals undergoing cancer treatment have shown that medical marijuana can help in managing the following:

Pain. Marijuana can work similarly to opioids (the strongest pain relievers available) when treating individuals living with cancer related pain. Additionally, it may have anti-inflammatory effects that can help with pain. Some treatment plans may include both opioids and marijuana.

Neuropathy. Neuropathy is a medical term for nerve damage, which is a common complication of chemotherapy and other cancer treatments. It is typically characterized by a feeling of weakness, numbness, tingling, or burning in the hands and feet. Medical marijuana has been shown to provide relief for those experiencing pain from neuropathy.

Nausea and vomiting. Many individuals living with cancer experience nausea and vomiting as a side effect of chemotherapy. There are many medications available to treat this symptom. Dronabinol is a synthetic cannabinoid that is approved by the U.S.

Food and Drug Administration (FDA) for this indication. Additionally, studies have shown that medical marijuana can be an effective treatment for nausea and vomiting.

Anorexia or cachexia. Anorexia is the medical term for loss of appetite. Cachexia and wasting syndrome is a phenomenon of unintentional weight loss, specifically the loss of lean muscle and fat. It is often accompanied by fatigue and a decline in functional abilities. The synthetic cannabinoid dronabinol is also FDA-approved for anorexia associated with acquired immune deficiency syndrome (AIDS), but not specifically for cancer. There are limited studies that demonstrate the efficacy of medical marijuana in the management of these symptoms. However, marijuana may improve one's appetite and this condition may be a state-approved indication for medical marijuana.

Anti-neoplastic. Pre-clinical studies (lab and animal testing) show that marijuana may be effective in slowing down or stopping the growth of certain tumors. To date, there has been one small human trial to study this anti-cancer effect. However, there are other studies that show an association between recreational marijuana use and the development of certain cancers. These studies do not show that marijuana is a cause of these cancers, but only that there could be some link. Further research is needed to understand the safety profile and potential anti-neoplastic effects of this treatment.

The labeling of marijuana as an illegal drug has greatly limited the research of its medical applications. However, there has been increasing interest in this field over the past few decades. More studies are needed to fully understand the exciting potential benefits to improve symptoms and quality of life for individuals living with cancer.

Questions to Ask Your Health Care Team

It is important to maintain open and honest communication with your health care team about any symptoms or pain that you are experiencing. This will help your health care team determine if medical marijuana is a treatment option for you. Here are a few questions you may want to ask your doctor when discussing if medical marijuana is appropriate for you:

Medical Marijuana and Cancer

What are the medical marijuana laws in the state I live in? Each state has different laws dictating qualifying conditions and dispensing of medical marijuana. Medical marijuana and patient ID cards should not be used or transported out of state, given that the legal status of marijuana varies state to state. For up-to-date state and federal laws.

How can I be certified to receive medical marijuana? Registered doctors and nurse practitioners can certify you to receive medical marijuana. Ask your doctor to you help you find a registered health care professional and about the certification process in your state.

Will smoking marijuana do more harm than good? There are many different ways to take medical marijuana, like pills, edibles, vaporization, oils, drops, topical, or a spray. If you and doctor are considering medical marijuana as a treatment option, it's important to discuss the best form for you according to the availability of products in your state.

What are the side effects of medical marijuana? Keep in mind that side effects can vary from person to person based on the product used. Medical marijuana can cause some side effects and drug interactions that should be discussed with your health care team. Some side effects include sleepiness, mood changes, decreased blood pressure, and changes in heart rate.

Cannabis And Cancer: How "Marijuana" Helps The Body Heal

The cannabis plant (also known as the hemp plant) has been used in just about every culture for centuries. In fact, cannabis is included in the 50 fundamental herbs within the cornucopia of Traditional Chinese Medicine. It has been cited in ancient texts as having a healing effect on over 100 ailments. Recently in the United States, the collective mood is changing in regards to cannabis/hemp (aka "marijuana").

Some peopled9x\ prefer to use the term "hemp" or "cannabis" since those are proper names for the plant, and the truth is that the term "marijuana" (derived from the Mexican slang "marihuana") was popularized in the early 1930s by the Federal Bureau of Narcotics (which later became the DEA) in order to make this amazing plant sound sinister and to elude the public's existing familiarity and comfort level with the plant and the medical application of cannabis/hemp tinctures. "Marijuana" was not a commonly smoked recreational drug at the time.

Currently there are 25 states where it is legal for patients to use "marijuana" for medical purposes. Pending federal legislation may open up opportunities for federally-funded medical research, including human clinical trials. This will further prove cannabis' track-record when it comes to healing a number of disease conditions including cancer.

Cannabis and The Endocannabinoid System

In the mid-1990s, renowned Israeli researcher Dr. Ralph Mechaoulam, professor of Medicinal Chemistry at Hebrew University in Jerusalem, made an exciting discovery that would forever change how we look at our biological relationship to plant medicine. Dr. Mechaoulam discovered a subtle system within the body that seemed to have a balancing effect on every other system. He called it the Endocannabinoid (EC) System and it can be found in all mammals, including humans.

The EC system consists of a series of molecular receptors that are designed to receive cannabinoids. In particular this includes cannabidiol (CBD) and tetrahydrocannabinol (THC) as well as other related substances such as cannabigerol (CBG) and cannabinol (CBN).

Prior research in the 1980s led Mechaoulam and others to pinpoint two main receptors for cannabinoids - cannabinoid 1 (CB1) and cannabinoid 2 (CB2). Researchers at the time also defined the natural substances called endocannabinoids, which our body produces on its own in a similar way it produces endorphins. Phytocannabinoids (namely THC, CBD, and their variants), on the other hand, come directly from the cannabis plant.

Cannabinoid receptors CB1 and CB2 are designed by the body to be specific targets for THC, while our natural endocannabinoids help to synthesize it. The process of THC-cannabinoid receptor binding and what this does for the body is what researchers have been studying for over two decades. They are doing this in order to find out exactly how cannabis works in healing cancer.

Microbiologist Dr. Christine Sanchez of Compultense Univeristy in Madrid, Spain has been studying cannabinoids and cancer since the early 2000s. She was the first to discover the antitumor effects of cannabinoids.

We now know that the endocannabinoid system regulates a lot of biological functions such as appetite, food intake, motor function, reproduction and many others and that is why the plant has such a wide therapeutic potential.

Cannabis and Cancer Tumor Growth

We observed that when we treated astrocytoma, a type of brain tumor cells with cannabinoids, the THC…was killing the cells in our Petri dishes," Dr. Sanchez says. "We…decided to analyze these components in animal models of breast and brain tumors. The results we are obtaining are telling us that cannabinoids may be useful for the treatment of Breast Cancer."

Sanchez and other researchers have confirmed that the most potent effects against tumor growth occur when THC and CBD are combined.

Cannabidiol, or CBD, which does not have a psychoactive effect, has long been known as a potent anti-cancer agent. This is because of its ability to interfere with cellular communication in tumors as well as in its ability to instigate apoptosis, or programmed cancer cell death. Some research studies, including in vitro and animal-based trials conducted by San Francisco-based researchers at the California Pacific Medical Center, have also shown that CBD may affect genes involved in aggressive metastasis. It does this by helping to shut down cellular growth receptors.

Tetrahydrocannabinol (i.e. THC), the psychoactive counterpart to CBD, has been shown to reduce tumor growth as well. It has also shown to have an effect on the rate of metastasis, including for non-small cell lung cancer - the leading cause of cancer deaths globally. A 2007 study on THC and highly-aggressive epidermal growth factor receptor-overexpressing (EGF-expressing) lung cancer conducted by Harvard Medical School found that certain EGF lung cancer cells express CB1 and CB2 cannabinoid receptors. They found that the presence of THC effected metastasis of these cells by reducing the "focal adhesion complex," which plays a vital role in cancer migration.

Studies have also been conducted on the combined effect of CBD and THC on lung, prostate, colon, pancreatic, liver, bladder, cervical, blood-based, brain, and other forms of cancer. These studies lend increasing evidence to the fact that cannabinoids are not only antioxidant phytonutrients but powerful "herbal chemo" agents.

Says Dr. Sanchez: "One of the advantages of cannabinoid-based medicines would be that they target specifically tumor cells. They don't have any toxic effect on normal non-tumoral cells. This is an advantage with respect to standard chemotherapy that targets basically everything."

If You Use Cannabis for Cancer, Do it Right

Because cannabinoid therapy is relatively new in the mainstream, a current challenge for patients regarding its use is lack of regulation. This may change, however, with the possible passing of the Compassionate Access, Research Expansion, and

Respect States (CARERS) Act, which has the support of 37 members of Congress.

CARERS would remove "marijuana" from the Controlled Substances Act Schedule I drug category, where it has been since 1970 - on par with heroin and cocaine. This classification is ridiculous since, by definition.

Think about it. How can HHS hold a medical use patent for cannabis oil if there are no medical uses for cannabis? OK, enough of the logic lesson. Let's just say that there are some serious logic deficiencies in these laws.

If "marijuana" is rightfully removed from a Schedule drug, this would open the door for more targeted, federally-funded research as well as increased patient access to this amazing healing plant.

In the meantime, if you are on a cancer-healing path and are considering using cannabinoids, here are some general guidelines that experts agree are worth considering:

Know your source. Unfortunately, because the medical cannabis industry is largely unregulated, charlatans selling bogus products definitely exist. You should not have to pay exorbitant amounts of money for any cannabis product that you buy from regulated pharmacies or online. Also, make quality a priority for you. Be sure that your product comes from an organic source and that you know that the plant has not been grown or processed using pesticides.

Stick with natural cannabis products. Synthetically-produced cannabinoids such as Marinol are commercially available. However, anecdotal evidence has found that these do not work as efficiently as natural substances do.

Work with a professional healthcare provider trained in cannabinoid therapy. These professionals are out there in increasing numbers, especially in states where the medical cannabis industry is well established or growing, such as California and Colorado. Reach out to a patient advocate group online if no qualified professionals are in your area.

Make cannabis therapy an important part of your overall cancer-healing toolbox. A well-rounded naturally-based cancer healing protocol involves working with the body's own healing mechanisms through a variety of means. For you, this may mean changes to your diet and lifestyle, reducing stress, getting quality sleep, moving your body, intense detoxing protocols, and using other supplements and proven natural methods in addition to the powerful healing power of cannabis.

Cancer: Can Cannabis Really Cure It?

Cancer is a disease that looms large. It is one of the leading causes of death and one in three of us will be diagnosed with it during our lifetimes. Unfortunately, the cancer rates are only rising. The National Institute of Cancer estimates that by 2030, its death toll will have increased by 60%. Some are looking to cannabis to cure this deadly disease. But is cannabis a cure – or is this just wishful thinking?

Cancer Patient Success Stories With Medical Pot

Anecdotal accounts abound of patients curing their

own cancer using high-potency edible cannabis extracts. Take Dennis Hill, a prostate cancer patient who decided to forgo chemotherapy and try cannabis instead. His story of complete recovery after six months of cannabis use is available online – along with his medical record and journal of his progress. Or Kelly Hauf – who decided to try cannabis oil in the months leading up to a scheduled surgery to remove a brain tumor. After eight months of treatment, there was nothing left of her tumor to remove. These stories are hard to ignore – but many doctors advise patients not to assume that cannabis was the cause of these incredible recoveries.

Doctors Cautious About Weed for Cancer

Dr. Abrams, a leading oncologist at the UCSF Osher Center for Integrative Medicine says he has seen cannabis help many with the side effects of cancer but cautions against assuming cannabis is a cure. He says given his high proportion of cannabis using patients, 'if cannabis definitively cured cancer, I would have expected that I would have a lot more survivors.'

Cannabis is well-established as a treatment for the side effects of cancer and chemotherapy, like nausea, vomiting, pain, anxiety, insomnia, and lack of appetite. But in a comprehensive review of the cannabis literature, researchers from the National Academies of Sciences, Engineering and Medicine found there to be insufficient evidence to say that cannabis can treat cancer directly. Without large-scale, placebo controlled clinical trials, doctors and researchers don't have the solid evidence they'd need to recommend cannabis for cancer treatment.

Science Shows Cannabis Has Anti-Cancer Properties

Still other scientists are more hopeful about cannabis'

potential efficacy, and point to laboratory and animal studies that show cannabinoids like CBD and THC kill cancer cells in laboratory conditions — without harming the healthy cells nearby. While clinical trials on human subjects is still a ways off — given cannabis' status as a controlled substance – the preclinical data gives reason to hope that patients stories of success aren't just flukes.

"There is a large body of scientific data which indicates that cannabinoids specifically inhibit cancer cell growth and promote cancer cell death" explains Dr. David Meiri, the lead researcher on an Israeli project studying 50 varieties of cannabis and its effects on 200 different cancer cells. Meiri and his team have successfully killed brain and breast cancer cells through exposure to cannabis and they are hopeful they can find more varieties of cancer cells that respond to this treatment.

Still, experts caution against forgoing traditional treatment options. Dr. Meiri's research suggests that not all cancer cells respond to cannabinoids in the same way. Even if cannabis can help with some cancers, it might not work the same for all. Additional research, specifically placebo-controlled clinical trials, are needed to fully understand how to handle each type of cancer individually.

With a condition as deadly as cancer, it is crucial to know whether a high cannabinoid regimen would work for any particular case, before foregoing alternatives that might help. Still while clinical research on cannabis continues to stall, patients must decide whether to wait indefinitely or follow in the footsteps of patients before them – experimenting with cannabis on their own.

Marijuana And Cancer

Marijuana is the name given to the dried buds and leaves of varieties of the Cannabis sativa plant, which can grow wild in warm and tropical climates throughout the world and be cultivated commercially. It goes by many names, including pot, grass, cannabis, weed, hemp, hash, marihuana, ganja, and dozens of others.

Marijuana has been used in herbal remedies for centuries. Scientists have identified many biologically active components in marijuana. These are called cannabinoids. The two best studied components are the chemicals delta-9-

tetrahydrocannabinol (often referred to as THC), and cannabidiol (CBD). Other cannabinoids are being studied.

At this time, the US Drug Enforcement Administration (DEA) lists marijuana and its cannabinoids as Schedule controlled substances. This means that they cannot legally be prescribed, possessed, or sold under federal law. Whole or crude marijuana (including marijuana oil or hemp oil) is not approved by the US Food and Drug Administration (FDA) for any medical use. But the use of marijuana to treat some medical conditions is legal under state laws in many states.

Dronabinol, a pharmaceutical form of THC, and a man-made cannabinoid drug called nabilone are approved by the FDA to treat some conditions.

Marijuana

Different compounds in marijuana have different actions in the human body. For example, delta-9-tetrahydrocannabinol (THC) seems to cause the "high" reported by marijuana users, and also can help relieve pain and nausea, reduce inflammation, and can act as an antioxidant. Cannabidiol (CBD) can help treat seizures, can reduce anxiety and paranoia, and can counteract the "high" caused by THC.

Different cultivars (strains or types) and even different crops of marijuana plants can have varying amounts of these and other active compounds. This means that marijuana can have different effects based on the strain used.

The effects of marijuana also vary depending on how marijuana compounds enter the body:

When taken by mouth, such as in baked goods, the THC is absorbed poorly and can take hours to be absorbed. Once it's absorbed, it's processed by the liver, which produces a second psychoactive compound (a substance that acts on the brain and changes mood or consciousness) that affects the brain differently than THC.

When marijuana is smoked or vaporized (inhaled), THC enters the bloodstream and goes to the brain quickly. The second psychoactive compound is produced in small amounts, and so has less effect. The effects of inhaled marijuana fade faster than marijuana taken by mouth.

How can marijuana affect symptoms of cancer?

A number of small studies of smoked marijuana found that it can be helpful in treating nausea and vomiting from cancer chemotherapy.

A few studies have found that inhaled (smoked or vaporized) marijuana can be helpful treatment of neuropathic pain (pain caused by damaged nerves).

Smoked marijuana has also helped improve food intake in HIV patients in studies.

There are no studies in people of the effects of marijuana oil or hemp oil.

Studies have long shown that people who took marijuana extracts in clinical trials tended to need less pain medicine.

More recently, scientists reported that THC and other cannabinoids such as CBD slow growth and/or cause death in certain types of cancer cells growing in lab dishes. Some animal studies also suggest certain cannabinoids may slow growth and reduce spread of some forms of cancer.

There have been some early clinical trials of cannabinoids in treating cancer in humans and more studies are planned. While the studies so far have shown that cannabinoids can be safe in treating cancer, they do not show that they help control or cure the disease.

Relying on marijuana alone as treatment while avoiding or delaying conventional medical care for cancer may have serious health consequences.

Possible harms of marijuana

Marijuana can also pose some harms to users. While the most common effect of marijuana is a feeling of euphoria ("high"), it also can lower the user's control over movement, cause disorientation, and sometimes cause unpleasant thoughts or feelings of anxiety and paranoia.

Smoked marijuana delivers THC and other cannabinoids to the body, but it also delivers harmful substances to users and those close by, including many of the same substances found in tobacco smoke.

Because marijuana plants come in different strains with different levels of active compounds, it can make each user's experience very hard to predict. The effects can also differ based on how deeply and for how long the user inhales. Likewise, the effects of ingesting marijuana orally can vary between people. Also, some chronic users can develop an unhealthy dependence on marijuana.

Cannabinoid drugs

There are 2 chemically pure drugs based on marijuana compounds that have been approved in the US for medical use.

Dronabinol (Marinol®) is a gelatin capsule containing delta-9-tetrahydrocannabinol (THC) that's approved by the US Food and Drug Administration (FDA) to treat nausea and vomiting caused by cancer chemotherapy as well as weight loss and poor appetite in patients with AIDS.

Nabilone (Cesamet®) is a synthetic cannabinoid that acts much like THC. It can be taken by mouth to treat nausea and vomiting caused by cancer chemotherapy when other drugs have not worked.

Nabiximols is a cannabinoid drug still under study in the US. It's a mouth spray made up of a whole-plant extract with THC and cannabidiol (CBD) in an almost one to one mix. It's available in Canada and parts of Europe to treat pain linked to cancer, as well as muscle spasms and pain from multiple sclerosis (MS). It's not approved in the US at this time, but it's being tested in clinical trials to see if it can help a number of conditions.

How can cannabinoid drugs affect symptoms of cancer?

Based on a number of studies, dronabinol can be helpful for reducing nausea and vomiting linked to chemotherapy.

Dronabinol has also been found to help improve food intake and prevent weight loss in patients with HIV. In studies of cancer patients, though, it wasn't better than placebo or another drug (megestrol acetate).

Nabiximols has shown promise for helping people with cancer pain that's unrelieved by strong pain medicines, but it hasn't been found to be helpful in every study done. Research is still being done on this drug.

Side effects of cannabinoid drugs

Like many other drugs, the prescription cannabinoids, dronabinol and nabilone, can cause side effects and complications.

Some people have trouble with increased heart rate, decreased blood pressure (especially when standing up), dizziness or lightheadedness, and fainting. These drugs can cause drowsiness as well as mood changes or a feeling of being "high" that some people find uncomfortable. They can also worsen depression, mania, or other mental illness. Some patients taking nabilone in studies reported hallucinations. The drugs may increase some effects of sedatives, sleeping pills, or alcohol, such as sleepiness and poor coordination. Patients have also reported problems with dry mouth and trouble with recent memory.

Older patients may have more problems with side effects and are usually started on lower doses.

People who have had emotional illnesses, paranoia, or hallucinations may find their symptoms are worse when taking cannabinoid drugs.

Talk to your doctor about what you should expect when taking one of these drugs. It's a good idea to have someone with you when you first start taking one of these drugs and after any dose changes.

What does the American Cancer Society say about the use of marijuana in people with cancer?

The American Cancer Society supports the need for more scientific research on cannabinoids for cancer patients, and recognizes the need for better and more effective therapies that can overcome the often debilitating side effects of cancer and its treatment. The Society also believes that the classification of marijuana as a Schedule controlled substance by the US Drug Enforcement Administration imposes numerous conditions on researchers and deters scientific study of cannabinoids. Federal officials should examine options consistent with federal law for enabling more scientific study on marijuana.

Medical decisions about pain and symptom management should be made between the patient and his or her doctor, balancing evidence of benefit and harm to the patient, the patient's preferences and values, and any laws and regulations that may apply.

The American Cancer Society Cancer Action Network (ACS CAN), the Society's advocacy affiliate, has not taken a position on legalization of marijuana for medical purposes because of the need for more scientific research on marijuana's potential benefits and harms. However, ACS CAN opposes the smoking or vaping of marijuana and other cannabinoids in public places because the carcinogens in marijuana smoke pose numerous health hazards to the patient and others in the patient's presence.

Everything We Know About Treating Anxiety With Weed

Weed can, for some, cause anxiety. This is one of the best-known bits of cannabis lore, and according to psychologist Susan Stoner (yes), who has reviewed the scientific literature on cannabis's effects on mental health, it's also one of the most commonly documented adverse effects of using pot or pot-based products.

At the same time, many in the cannabis community believe, weed can also help people to treat or manage their anxiety. Faith in this paradox is so widespread—and anxiety is such a common issue—

that research psychologist Carrie Cuttler recently found "it was the number two reason medical cannabis patients reported using cannabis.

Is there research on weed and anxiety?

As with other common claims about weed's purported benefits, though, most of the people who've researched cannabis and its components believe it's too soon to say whether or not they can actually help with anxiety. "There is little research evidence on the effects of cannabis in treating anxiety," Cuttler says, "or on the doses and strains that may be most beneficial." Future research could nail down clear and effective weed-based treatments for at least some kinds of anxiety or some people.

Common narratives hold that many weed-based anxiety stories stem from inexperienced users blindsided by the sensation of being high. More generally, though, the story goes that stressed brains often have cannabinoid shortages, so a little weed just evens things out. The relaxing effects of a good high can also help to cut down on the symptoms of a bout of acute stress.

Is a high CBD or THC strain better for anxiety?

Some people may feel anxious when smoking pot even as they gain experience because everyone reacts differently to it; these folks should just stay away from weed. But for everyone else, publications like High Times and Leafly regularly recommend particular strains they claim will help with various types of anxiety—often those heavier on soothing CBD than on high-inducing THC.

Existing research aligns with common wisdom and recommendations to a degree. We know, for instance, that THC and CBD—major components of weed—interact with systems in the brain that influence anxiety. THC can work on these systems to reduce anxiety in some people at low doses, but the risk of tripping over to anxious responses gets higher with higher doses.

A few studies, meanwhile, suggest that CBD has more general and reliable anti-anxiety effects. The mechanisms by which each of these substances affects anxiety remain a little murky. Still, this all seems to support the idea that "a higher ratio of THC to CBD is more likely to cause anxiety," says Carl Stevenson, a neuroscientist who has researched the effects of compounds within cannabis on fear and anxiety, "while a lower ratio may have the opposite effect—relieving anxiety."

However, research on cannabis and its effects on anxiety is entirely embryonic. Most of what we know is based on animal models, which neuroscientist and cannabis researcher Ryan McLaughlin stresses do not always translate well into humans. The few human studies that have been done, adds anxiety disorder researcher Michael van Ameringen, have been small and limited in their scope and methodologies. They have usually only explored healthy populations, not people with clear and defined anxiety disorders in clinical settings, and definitely not over long-term periods.

There's anxiety that's acute versus chronic. There's anxiety that has a more strongly traumatic aspect to it," like PTSD. Different forms of anxiety may have slightly different neurochemical roots, leading to different cannabis-linked effects. Cannabis may also only affect some elements of anxiety rather than the whole condition; van Ameringen stresses, for instance, that while studies seem to show weed-based products may help people with PTSD sleep and avoid flashbacks, it may not help, and could even worsen, their overall conditions. On top of that, Stoner notes, every individual could have different reactions to cannabis and the compounds within it based on their genetics or even the cultural messaging they've internalized about how a given substance should affect them.

As of now, researchers do not know with any certainty what forms or aspects of anxiety THC or CBD might be able to help with in general or in specific populations. Nor do they know if these or other compounds might trigger anxiety or exacerbate anxiety disorders in certain populations.

The unknowns get even more extreme when we talk about whole plant cannabis versus specific compounds isolated from it. There are more than 100 other cannabinoids in the average pot leaf, McLaughlin notes, not to mention other potentially important compounds like terpenes. "We know almost nothing about these compounds. We certainly do not know if any of the effects" cannabis users have reported over the years "are attributed to interactions between" them.

What kind of strain or weed products should I buy to help treat anxiety?

"All in all," Stoner says, "it is practically pure speculation what any given strain or product might do to any particular person with regard to anxiety." That's especially true when one considers how unreliable the quality or contents of a given strain might be from store to store or batch to batch, and how many other elements might be in something sold as, say, a pure CBD supplement.

Current or prospective cannabis users interested in anxiety management don't often hear about these nuances or limitations because so much information circulating in dispensaries and online is based on anecdotes or personal experiences. When cannabis resources engage with existing studies, Stoner argues, they often oversimplify and misrepresent them as well. Some resources and retailers do a good job of exercising caution and offering solid, nuanced advice, notes Giordano. But for potential customers it can be difficult to tell who those reliable brokers are.

Until the research advances to the point that we can speak more definitively about the intersections of cannabis, its constituent compounds, and anxiety—which could take quite some time given pot's legal status, our current level of knowledge, and funding issues—most researchers recommend that people look elsewhere for help with their anxiety. Van Ameringen points out there are plenty of effective medications for anxiety. For those who don't want to be dependent on pills, Cuttler adds that short-term cognitive behavioral therapy and similar treatments can be quite effective for managing many types of short- and long-term anxiety.

What should I do if I'm still going to take weed for anxiety?

For anyone who hasn't had success with these treatments, or who is set on exploring weed for anxiety management, the researchers I've spoken to have a few pieces of advice: Given what we know thus far, they recommend using a high-CBD or CBD-only product—at least something with equal parts CBD and THC. McLaughlin notes that, so long as we lack definitive scientific evidence, anecdotal info about ideal strains can be useful, but should not be taken as gospel. Careful experimentation with different strains is a must. As with any new drug,

Giordano recommends starting with a low dose and moving up slowly; Cuttler recommends methodically noting any changes in symptom and experience to get a sense of what's working and what isn't.

If you find something that does work for whatever type of anxiety you're experiencing, that's great. But Cuttler advises against relying on it as a long-term solution. The limited research we have suggests that people can develop tolerances to pot or related products' useful effects, and may even develop negative side effects, perhaps even worsening their anxiety, over the long-term.

None of this is likely what those seeking relief from their anxiety through weed or a weed-based product want to hear. Unfortunately this is just the state of weed science right now: provisional at best and often misrepresented. Until that changes, it's better to approach weed-based solutions with due caution.

Medical Marijuana And Anxiety Disorders

Whether you just received a diagnosis or have grappled with it for years, anxiety can be very difficult to deal with. Regardless of the severity of your case, an anxiety disorder makes usually simple activities feel like insurmountable tasks.

Some patients have difficulty finding the right treatment for their anxiety. Since we all have unique brain chemistry and react differently to anxiety meds, the same treatment won't affect every patient in the same way. In addition to this, finding the right therapist adds another layer to the confusion.

As we learn more about medical marijuana, we are continually discovering new ways it can serve as a natural alternative to pharmaceutical medicine. There is increasing evidence showing medical marijuana can be an effective treatment for anxiety disorders. To help answer any questions you might have, we'll go over the basics of medical marijuana as a treatment for anxiety disorders, so you can decide whether or not it might be an option for you.

About Anxiety Disorders

Anxiety disorders include a wide range of mental illnesses such as:

Generalized anxiety disorder (GAD) — People with GAD experience frequent and excessive nervousness about many facets of everyday life and have a hard time controlling these worries. Even when they know they're experiencing more anxiety than is warranted for a situation, they can't stop feeling concerned.

Obsessive-compulsive disorder (OCD) — While most people think of OCD as being overly neat or organized, it causes as much distress as other anxiety disorders. OCD causes intrusive thoughts — or obsessions — that compel the patient to conduct repeated actions — or compulsions — to calm down.

Social anxiety disorder — Another misunderstood form of anxiety, social anxiety disorder, goes far beyond shyness. In reality, it makes the patient feel severe anxiety about social interaction. They often worry about judgment from others when in social situations.

Panic disorder — Patients with panic disorder get sudden, unpredicted panic attacks that cause a racing heartbeat, hyperventilation and other intense symptoms. They often worry about getting panic attacks, which compounds the issue.

Post-traumatic stress disorder (PTSD) — Patients who have gone through a traumatic event, such as war, disasters, abuse, tragedy or other life-changing or life-threatening occurrences, can develop PTSD. This illness causes the patient to have intense flashbacks about the event, avoid trauma reminders and constantly feel on edge.

Specific phobias — We all have our fears, but patients with phobias have an extreme fear reaction to the thing they are afraid of. Even though they know they have an irrational fear, they have difficulty controlling it.

Like other mental illness patients, people with anxiety disorders are often dismissed as overreacting. Sometimes, people will tell them just to calm down.

But people with anxiety have a much harder time calming down than someone without it.

Most people have to make a living by working, getting an education, taking care of their household or serving another important purpose. Regardless of your goal in life, constant anxiety impairs your ability to meet it.

But there is hope. Your feelings of anxiety are valid. We're here to give you support for your medical marijuana treatment, and there are many professionals out there who can help you feel better.

Symptoms of Anxiety Disorders

Anxiety disorders can cause many symptoms that interfere with your everyday functioning, including:

- Episodes of severe anxiety or fear that cause intense reactions like sweating, rapid heartbeat, shortness of breath, nausea or sweating

- Racing or pounding heartbeat

- Feelings of apprehension or dread

- Shortness of breath

- Insomnia

- Restlessness

- Fatigue

- Inability to concentrate

The combination of symptoms you have and their intensity can vary depending on the nature of your anxiety disorder. Just because you don't experience these exact symptoms doesn't mean you don't have an anxiety disorder — only an experienced mental health professional can provide a proper diagnosis.

Typical Treatments for Anxiety Disorders

Treatments for anxiety disorders often take a multidisciplinary approach. The two primary types of anxiety treatment are:

Cognitive behavioral therapy (CBT) This is also known as "talk therapy," and it involves regular sessions with a licensed therapist where you talk about your feelings and behaviors. CBT focuses on addressing your negative and false beliefs and finding ways to manage them. For example, an anxiety patient might talk about their fears and worries to work towards rethinking them.

Medication — Doctors may also prescribe medication to reduce your anxiety symptoms. If you only have issues with anxiety, they will prescribe an anti-anxiety medication. But if you also have depression, some antidepressants also help anxiety.

Medical Marijuana as a Substitute for Anti-Anxiety Medication

The information we have about medical marijuana suggests that it could act as a replacement for typical anti-anxiety medication. Preliminary research about medical marijuana and anxiety shows cannabis has similar components to manufactured pharmaceuticals for anxiety symptoms.

One of the most commonly prescribed types of anti-anxiety medication is benzodiazepines. It manages the levels of a neurotransmitter called GABA that balances your anxiety levels. Unfortunately, patients who take them tend to build a tolerance quickly, and they cause thousands of overdose deaths every year.

Medical marijuana also shows potential for lowering your levels of cortisol, a hormone that indicates how much stress you feel. The lowered cortisol creates a dulled reaction to stress. We aren't quite sure whether this is an overall good or bad result yet, but this effect could be a total game-changer if it does turn out to be positive.

Using Medical Cannabis for Anxiety Disorder Symptoms

Medical marijuana can serve as a holistic alternative to anxiety medication without the typical side effects. It has been an effective treatment for symptoms of anxiety disorders for countless patients just like you.

However, some patients experience an increase in anxiety when they use cannabis meds. Don't worry, though with consultation from a marijuana doctor and care in picking the right strain, you can avoid the extra anxiety.

The cannabis compound known as CBD has been shown to offer substantial benefits for people suffering from a variety of anxiety disorders. Cannabis that is rich in CBD has been used in patients who were suffering from anxiety as well as pain, spasms and many other issues. You can't get high from CBD, and it offers several therapeutic effects.

Research into the benefits of medical cannabis for anxiety is still in its early stages, but indications show that marijuana can help people suffering from anxiety a great deal.

However, we should also keep in mind that marijuana has the potential to cause psychosis that triggers anxiety. As marijuana laws change, we'll be able to have more opportunities for research that can tell us when and how to properly use marijuana for anxiety. In the meantime, we recommend working closely with your doctor so you can figure out whether or not it works for you.

Best Strains of Medical Cannabis for Anxiety Disorders

When you get your cannabis meds, you must choose a strain that suits your health needs. Medicating with marijuana isn't as simple as getting any kind of leaf and using it — every strain of marijuana has unique effects. But it isn't terribly complicated as long as you do your research and consult with your doctor and dispensary.

Before we talk about specific strains, keep in mind that there are two families of strains — Indica and Sativa. Indica is high in CBD, the chemical in marijuana beneficial for anxiety, while Sativa has

THC, which can cause anxiety. So you'll want to find an Indica or Indica-leaning hybrid that has a high amount of CBD.

One Can Conclude

Marijuana is a green or gray mixture of dried, shredded flowers and leaves of the hemp plant Cannabis sativa. The main active chemical in marijuana is THC (delta-9-tetrahydrocannabinol). The membranes of certain nerve cells contain protein receptors that bind THC, kicking off a series of cellular reactions that ultimately lead to the high that users experience when they smoke marijuana.

More than half of U.S. states and the District of Columbia have legalized medical marijuana in some form, and more are considering bills to do the same. Yet while many people are using marijuana for effective treatments, the FDA still hasn't approved it as a treatment for illnesses because there haven't been enough studies to prove that it's safe and effective. My hope is for scientist, doctors and researchers continue to work and come up with conclusive evidence that will lead to FDA approvals for drugs related to Cannabis.

If you received any value in this book would you do the favor of leaving a book review. Thank you and God bless you.

www.ingramcontent.com/pod-product-compliance
Lightning Source LLC
Chambersburg PA
CBHW050555300426
44112CB00013B/1935